I0492751

Table of Contents

Cure (Not Just Manage) Irritable Bowel Syndrome: A Personal Narrative of Success

Written by

Catherine Mary Allen

UPDATED July 18, 2018 BY CATHERINE MARY ALLEN
© 2013, 2018 HGDG Arts All rights reserved

Contact: hgdgarts@gmail.com
HGDG Arts
Self-Healing Book Series
USA

All rights are reserved. Any information excerpted should credit this author by name in a citation or footnote and mention the author's full name and title of book along with a page reference where the info is located. Direct quotes should be indicated with quotation marks and paraphrased info should be cited. Any reviews on amazon.com are welcome. If you want a review copy, please email the publisher HGDGarts@gmail.com with details.

Introduction

In 1978, I was a school bus driver, separated after a failed marriage, and living in Texas. I took the train to Mexico City for a brief holiday and while there became ill with flu-like symptoms. I mistakenly drank the water in a downtown hotel. It was tap water which I believed to be safe bottled water. This was the start of a condition that doctors diagnosed as Irritable Bowel Syndrome (IBS). I suffered with this vacillating condition for decades. At age 51, I promised myself I would cure it and live a normal life. Two years later, I cured my IBS and have been symptom free for 19 years. I can assure you that my bowels act and react normally to anything and everything in my life, whether it is stress, emotional upset, food, or drink. I found a few things in my quest to cure myself that I'd like to share with anyone who suffers from IBS and seeks a cure, once and for all.

This book includes an update about five years after I first published the first Kindle book. The major point is that the functional chocolates I bought and used are no longer in business. There are other brands, though, that you will find in health food stores and possibly on vitacost.com.

IBS Diagnosis and Symptoms

With the first diagnosis of IBS in 1983, a nurse practitioner informed me that the positive side of having the mainly diarrhea form of the disease is that I would not get colon cancer since the stool did not sit in the colon long enough to cause problems. This may or may not be true, but since they found no indications of other problems in my stool samples, they told me I could manage the disease by diet and practicing relaxation techniques. This will probably sound familiar to any of you with IBS. Most doctors consider this motility issue in the bowel as one related to food allergies, food triggers, environmental factors, and psychological as well as physical stress.

In retrospect now, as I update my original book on my IBS cure, I believe the illness caused by drinking bad water in Mexico created a disease in my bowels that doctors did not discover through stool samples because it was several years after I was infected. The changed environment left my bowels weak and lacking in the what was physically needed for optimum function. Doctors treat symptoms with drugs and tell patients to avoid stressors that will strain the depleted bowels to avoid flare ups of symptoms. However, my cure came about because I replenished what was depleted through the Mexico illness making my bowels strong again. Finding this cure was trial and error on my part since doctors say it can't be cured, only managed. They are wrong.

Like others with IBS, I managed my IBS over the years to avoid embarrassing and unpredictable flare-ups. I quit drinking coffee with caffeine and eating spicy foods, for the most part. Eventually, I quit smoking cigarettes, too. Unfortunately, I also had a sweet tooth. One sure-fire trigger that immediately sent me running desperately to the bathroom was eating a donut and drinking a cup of coffee. It only took a few minutes after I ate and drank them for the urge to evacuate to take over. I had two to four minutes at most to reach a bathroom before I would be embarrassed with an accident of wet stool in my pants. If I did not already have digested food in my lower intestines from a meal eaten earlier, there would be nothing to worry about.

When I had IBS, the normal transit time for a meal to make it through my digestive system was half of the healthy normal 24-hour cycle. If I ate small quantities at meals, my digestive system would be less sensitive to triggers. However, even without specific triggers, like sugar and caffeine, stress, and strenuous or continuous exercise, I never had solid stools since the water-borne infection in Mexico City in 1978. Prior to that, I had normal and regular bowel movements, perfectly formed stools, and did not suffer from constipation or diarrhea, no matter what I ate or how much I had to eat or drink. Afterwards, even with periods when I had regularly timed bowel movements, usually in the morning after waking up, the stool was very loose (what doctors called "softserve" on The Doctors TV show) to stringy/mucous-textured/watery. It rushed out noisily at best to violently at the worst. I only passed a normal solid or hardened stool a few times in decades, and this was during rare instances of constipation when I had not passed a stool in days and needed castor oil to help pass it.

The medical professionals I saw to help with the condition had varying suggestions about the causes for flare-ups and how to lessen the frequency of flare-ups. Nevertheless, I lived with the condition for over twenty years managing to lessen symptoms by eliminating what one doctor along the way suggested: "Quit drinking coffee, smoking cigarettes, and eating white sugar sweets, and your IBS will go away." He said it arrogantly. When I eventually quit smoking cigarettes, drank only decaffeinated coffee, and cut out white sugary sweets, my IBS was still there. That arrogant medical doctor's so-called cure for IBS was not a cure at all even though it is indisputably better for anyone's overall health to eliminate some of these bad habits.

When I was thirty-five, another doctor suggested I was going through early menopause and fluctuating hormones were the cause of flare-ups. Another said that eating too many salads without bread to solidify the raw vegetables caused the constant soupy stools. However, even when I ate solid foods, the IBS symptoms never completely disappeared. My morning stools were watery, soupy, or the texture of soft-serve ice cream. Sometimes, I had two or three bowel movements per day. Flare-ups did not lessen or get worse based on which time of the month it was for my menstrual cycles, either. Despite this doctor's guess about the cause of my IBS, I was not going through early menopause.

Over the decades, there were studies and drugs being developed to help manage the symptoms of IBS and to calm down or normalize overactive or constipated bowels. I did not want to take prescription drugs for my symptoms because I had a fundamental distrust of pharmaceuticals. Since they were not a cure nor even guaranteed to eliminate the uncertainty and embarrassment that sudden bowel urgency caused, I did not think they were worth the costs and risks. Instead, I searched for natural remedies that could help IBS.

Searching for a Cure While
Living With IBS

Eventually, after menopause at age 51 (not age 35 as that one doctor suggested), I made a commitment to research the illness on my own and to try anything and everything I could to cure myself. I had nothing to lose adopting this attitude since medical professionals still had no cure for IBS. Menopause for women is a great time to reevaluate life and change habits, to rehabilitate old negatives as the body changes. As I wrote earlier, the fluctuation of hormones never much affected my IBS during my menstrual cycles or after they stopped. I knew that there was a fundamental malfunction in the bowels and digestive system that had not cleared up since the original Mexico infection in 1978.

First, 2002 was not the first year I began trying alternative therapies or other practices that were supposed to manage IBS symptoms, but that year I made up my mind to actually cure myself. Let me first review the many things I tried over the decades since my diagnosis that may or may not have helped to eventually cure me decades later. I would feel remiss if I did not mention my entire journey of and the things that did help to minimize symptoms, at least temporarily. Some may sound radical or off the wall, and they could have helped in some small way. I have always been willing to try natural remedies and treatments and consulted a naturopathic doctor (ND), homeopathic practitioners, and herbalists during the 1980s. There were many in Austin, Texas, where I lived at the time as part of the New Age culture that flourished in the area. Perhaps you tried some of these alternative therapies yourself.

To begin, let me go back to around 1979 when I stopped drinking alcoholic beverages. I am a very emotional artistic type and believe that psychological and emotional states contribute to physical disease. This is the fundamental principle behind Bach Flower Remedies[1]. The first time an herbalist gave me a combination of three Bach remedies at Herbs, Etc., a little herb shop in Austin, I felt as if a dark cloud lifted and the weight was lifted off my shoulders. I took eight drops three times a day from a 1 oz. dropper bottle, and the emotional relief continued.

When I had separated from my first husband at the time, I tried to ignore the emotional toll this major life event took on my life. It was then I started drinking nightly. Drinking was a habit I picked up from my husband, but it continued after the separation as a way to get back into a social life as a single woman. It was a bad habit, but coincidentally, I quit drinking a few months after finishing the Bach Flower dropper bottle. Whether this change is a direct result or part of a placebo effect, I can't say. Nevertheless, the facts indicate some sort of sequential correlation. My self-esteem was restored, too, even after the divorce from my first husband was finalized.

---

[1] http://www.bachflower.com/

I have always liked to walk and ride bicycles, so my exercise level remained about the same throughout my life. I started meditating a little, too, around this time, and the IBS symptoms were minimal. Flare-ups had specific strong triggers like ingesting a donut with coffee. I did not have to worry too much about sudden and uncontrollable urges unless I ate a large portion of spicy Mexican food or other specific triggers. I met my lifelong love and moved in with the man who would eventually become my second husband, Janek. He was five years younger than me and an aspiring professional musician. We maintained a romantic life as creative people leading a relatively healthy lifestyle. Still, my IBS was not cured. It was maintained and subdued most of the time.

Periodically, a sudden urge would create panic in me when I was in public. For example, I would be shopping and get the urge to defecate and have to rush to the public restroom in the store to relieve myself immediately. If someone else was in the restroom, I tried to wait so that the noise of my loose bowel movements did not embarrass me. Also, my noisy and loose bowel movements always smelled terribly. Often, I could not wait until I was alone in the restroom, so I flushed during the movement to masquerade the noise of the gas and liquid movement, and then again right after to flush away the smell as quickly as possible. These tactics did not fool those in the restroom with me. I always waited until everyone else left the restroom before exiting the stall to avoid even more embarrassment.

I suppose I was pretty lucky when the unexpected urge to defecate came since I almost always made it to a restroom. If I were driving, I would pull into a fast food restaurant or gas station and run to their public bathroom, almost always just in the nick of time. When I was hiking or taking my regular constitutional, which is what I called my walk around the neighborhood, I had to duck in somewhere out of sight when the unexpected urge came. I recall once having to squat in someone's open garage behind a pile of boxes. Another time, I had to squat in the middle of thick hedges bordering an industrial business parking lot hoping no one would see me. The fortunate thing about my IBS is that defecation was fast, so these stealthy moments of relief were over quickly minimizing, at least, the chances of being discovered. I always carried tissues with me no matter where I went and what I was doing—just in case.

Another habit I developed was to not eat or eat minimally while traveling or visiting with friends and relatives. No one but my husband and doctors knew I had IBS because I was embarrassed by it all. After reading about some of these personal situations I encountered because of the disease, you will understand why I would want to keep it a secret. It is an extremely embarrassing and debilitating situation that causes the sufferer to sneak, hide, cover up, avoid, restrict, and minimize the enjoyment of life's pleasures due to the ever-present unexpected urges that can show up at any time. I had to clean the spattered toilet every time I used it because of the wet and sometimes violent evacuation. I'm not certain whether my friends and relatives suspected this awful condition had become a way of life for me since defecation is a daily event.

Alternative Treatments I Tried Along the Way
That Did Not Cure Me

Experimenting with new natural treatments was part of my existence with IBS. Most did not cure IBS. At best, they helped to minimize some symptoms for a short a period of time. Some of the treatments and practices I tried over the years included the following:

- Ingesting an edible hydrogen peroxide and bacteriacide
- Ingesting aloe vera
- Doing a month-long bowel cleanse
- Taking colostrum
- Eating probiotic pills themselves
- Drinking buttermilk/eating yogurt
- Taking probiotics capsules alone
- Taking fiber
- Vegetarianism
- Drinking mint tea and taking calming herbs
- Avoiding red meat
- Boycotting sugar-free products with xylitol
- Avoiding gluten
- Switching to decaffeinated coffee and beverages

While this list of practices and treatments helped to mitigate some symptoms for short periods of time, they were not a cure, and I never had a normal, well-formed solid stool for decades. My bowel movements were always liquid or soft piles, at best, and mostly smelly because the food was not fully digested/processed, as well as usually noisy when coming out. Most of the practices listed above can help anyone's health, but none of them cured my IBS.

Additionally, I noticed that when I went to the dentist and had to take antibiotics like penicillin, my bowels settled down a little like they did after I took the non-prescription edible hydrogen peroxide and bactericide from the Naturapath. While the doctors I went to could not pinpoint a cause for my IBS, I knew it coincided with my trip to Mexico and the flu-like illness I contracted from drinking the tap water. I researched what sort of water-borne illnesses could be contracted in Mexico, and I thought it could be giardia, which eats away at the surface lining of the intestines. This is what I read about giardia, but I have no proof I was ever infected by giardia. Because the symptoms caused by the IBS were really rather ghastly to witness and live with, I feared permanent structural damage occurred to my intestines that could never be reversed.

Successful Self-Treatments that Work to Cure IBS

All I wanted was to have normal bowel movements and live my life freely without worry of embarrassment and constant restrictions to manage my IBS. As you who suffer with IBS know, management techniques do not assure freedom from symptoms, so I always had to be on guard and think twice before traveling away from home. Finally, I tried two new things that changed my life forever. I added these two major cures to the habit of taking one or two psyllium fiber capsules daily. Psyllium fiber capsules are easier to take than Metamucil for me since I did not like drinking Metamucil. You have to make sure you take the capsules with at least 6 ounces of water or other liquids. I used the Target brand because it was economical and easy to pick up at the local store.

Of course, taking fiber daily is a good habit anyway, especially when you eat sugary sweets because it helps the body to process the sugar when you ingest fiber with it. But this alone did not cure my IBS.

First Major Breakthrough – Functional Dark Chocolates with Probiotics

The first major item I found that made a huge difference was a probiotic put into dark chocolate. I read that chocolate helps the beneficial bacteria in probiotics travel to the lower intestines. Most other foods with beneficial bacteria like yogurt stay in the upper intestines, especially buttermilk bacteria. Even the probiotic capsules I took at one point did not travel throughout the entire digestive system alive. I received almost immediate relief when I ate this chocolate. I found it at Walgreens, and it was a little pricey for dark chocolate squares, but I tried it when it went on sale. I'm very happy I did. It tastes delicious if you like dark chocolate, but it also has an abundance of live probiotics in it. It is worth every penny.

It was no longer sold at Walgreens, and I had to buy Maramor chocolates with probiotics directly from the company online at maramor.com. This statement is true:

> Mary Ellen Sanders, executive director of the International Scientific Association of Probiotics and Prebiotics, said chocolate is a suitable vehicle for the organisms commonly called probiotics because the bacteria survive well in chocolate's high-fat environment.[2]

They were also sold at health food stores like GNC or Whole Foods in your area for about $15 a package containing 10 chocolates.

---

[2] http://www.dispatch.com/content/stories/business/2010/08/20/healthy-indulgence.html

Figure 1 – Chocolates I actually used

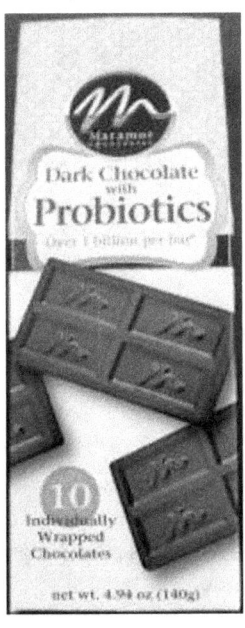

While this item is no longer available, there are now many other companies and brands selling probiotic chocolates since I first wrote this book. A google search using "probiotic chocolates" showed the following partial list. There are so many more brands selling this important product now. The image Figure 2 below shows the variety you will pull up if you search online.

Figure 2 – Google search sample for "probiotic chocolates"

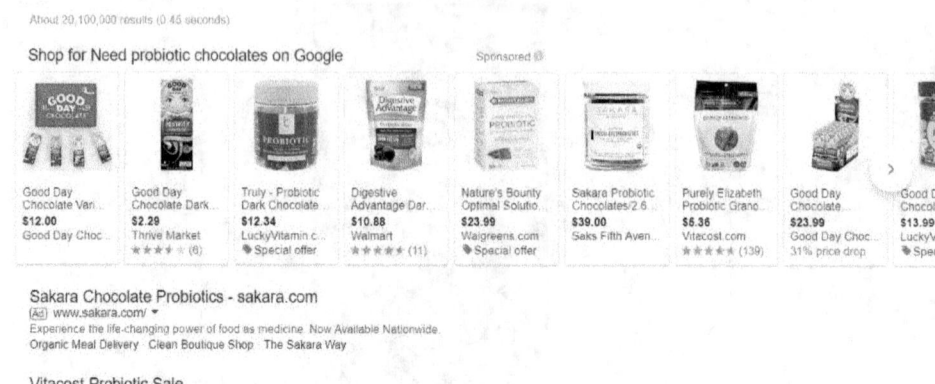

About 20,100,000 results (0.45 seconds)

Shop for Need probiotic chocolates on Google   Sponsored ⓘ

Good Day Chocolate Vari...	Good Day Chocolate Dark...	Truly - Probiotic Dark Chocolate	Digestive Advantage Dar...	Nature's Bounty Optimal Solutio...	Sakara Probiotic Chocolates/2.6...	Purely Elizabeth Probiotic Grano...	Good Day Chocolate...	Good Day Chocolate
$12.00	$2.29	$12.34	$10.88	$23.99	$39.00	$5.36	$23.99	$13.99
Good Day Choc...	Thrive Market	LuckyVitamin c...	Walmart	Walgreens.com	Saks Fifth Aven...	Vitacost.com	Good Day Choc...	LuckyVitam...
★★★★☆ (6)		♦ Special offer	★★★★☆ (11)	♦ Special offer		★★★★☆ (139)	31% price drop	♦ Special

Sakara Chocolate Probiotics - sakara.com
Ad www.sakara.com/ ▼
Experience the life-changing power of food as medicine. Now Available Nationwide.
Organic Meal Delivery · Clean Boutique Shop · The Sakara Way

Vitacost Probiotic Sale
Ad www.vitacost.com/Probiotics ▼
Get Up To 45% Off Probiotical Assortment Of Probiotics On Sale. Brands: Bluebonnet Nutrition,
Garden of Life, New Chapter, NOW Foods, Megafood, Jarrow Formulas.

Dark Chocolate: A Probiotic Food With Impressive Health Benefits

This image shows the many varieties and brands of probiotic chocolates available today. Choose wisely.

Even though some of these could be expensive, the brand I used helped to cure me of IBS after a few months by spreading beneficial bacteria throughout my entire digestive system all the way through the large colon. I can't recommend any of these individual brands since I used the brand I showed you and not these. These others if a reputable company should work. The key is to get one with dark chocolate and a high count of live probiotic bacteria.

I started taking one individually wrapped square a day for a few weeks and noticed a change in the next few days. My bowel movement did not have a large circumference, but it was solid and well formed. I assumed the diameter of the stool was so narrow because my intestines passed nothing but liquid and soft stools for so many decades. My stools tended to be on the narrow side at first. They are always well-formed and never liquid or soft. After a while of normal bowel movements, my stools were normally wide. I took the chocolates daily for a few weeks, and then I started eating them once or twice a week. I then ate them once in a while for boosters or after taking antibiotics. My bowels have never reverted to IBS symptoms ever again.

I suppose you can make your own probiotic chocolates by adding probiotic powder into melted dark chocolate being careful not to kill the beneficial bacteria by adding the probiotic powder when the chocolate is not too hot. I never tried this, but when I could no longer find the product at Walgreens, I thought I would have to make my own. Fortunately, I found them online and ordered that way instead. Now, you must either make your own probiotic dark chocolate or find them in health food or sports stores, etc. I do enjoy eating dark chocolate with yogurt for a snack, and this could also help to cure, but since I no longer have IBS, I can't verify that this can effectively cure you by delivering probiotics throughout the colon and entire digestive tract like functional dark chocolates did for me.

Today, June 23, 2018, I read about the beneficial effect of flavanols in good dark chocolate on

ConsumeLab.com and how helpful these chocolate flavanols are for bowel disease or discomfort. I wish a study on IBS sufferers using dark chocolates with probiotics along with the other item/s that worked for me would be conducted to help IBS patients cure their disease once and for all.

The Second Major Element That Helped to Cure My IBS – L-Glutamine

Another major supplement I took that cured my IBS was L-Glutamine. I bought one bottle of the NOW brand capsules on amazon.com.[3]

Glutamine has recently been the focus of much scientific interest. A growing body of evidence suggests that during certain stressful times, the body may require more Glutamine than it can produce. Under these circumstances Glutamine may be considered a "conditionally essential" amino acid. Glutamine is involved in maintaining a positive nitrogen balance (an anabolic state) and also aids rapidly growing cells (immune system lymphocytes and intestinal cell enterocytes). In addition, Glutamine is a

---

[3] http://www.amazon.com/NOW-Foods-L-Glutamine-500mg-Capsules/dp/B000QVCAKQ

regulator of acid-base balance and a nitrogen transporter.

L-Glutamine is an essential amino acid that is often given to cancer patients who have had radiation treatment for colon cancer because it aids in rebuilding the cell wall lining of the intestines. My logic in taking this supplement was what I read about giardia eating away the surface lining of the intestines making it difficult to process digested foods since beneficial bacteria could not establish themselves well. I took a 500 mg. capsule daily as directed and felt a difference in regularity and reliability. I only took a capsule occasionally every few months, later, especially after an illness like the flu or food poisoning, for maintenance. NOW brand L-Glutamine costs about $9 for 120 500mg. capsules, but any good source will do.

Figure 3 – This was an essential for my cure.

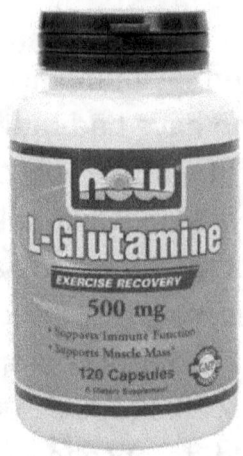

I used this brand and a few others for about 6 months and then as needed for a few years after antibiotics, etc., at the dentist, etc. Now, I don't really keep them on hand anymore.

Like the functional chocolates, I continued to take L-Glutamine occasionally after an illness or antibiotic treatment and had them on hand for a while after IBS stopped. The only daily supplement I took were the fiber capsules, about one per day and two or more when I eat sugary sweets. After I was confident that my IBS would never return about six years ago, I stopped taking these things, even after antibiotic treatment, etc., but I do enjoy yogurt and buttermilk as snacks anyway.

Today in 2018, I live a normal life trying to maintain a healthy eating pattern for my age. My stools are always normal and regular. They don't have an exceptionally terrible smell or make explosive noises coming out. I'm proud of my bowel movements today and even announce them jokingly to my husband some mornings because I cured myself of IBS after so many years of suffering.

My Healthy Life Without IBS

I have now lived IBS free for over a decade, and I don't have to worry about traveling and visiting friends for fear of an embarrassing accident. I drink strong coffee, Starbucks Espresso Roast, about 3 cups in the morning and more through the day sometimes. I don't like to eat breakfast all the time, so the coffee is how I start my day. Sometimes, I'll eat a sweet cake with my coffee, and my bowels react like anyone else's who has a normal, healthy digestive tract. I love spicy foods and enjoy Mexican salsas and jalapenos with no problems. I eat cayenne, black pepper, and other hot spices with any type of food I choose.

There was a time when I could not even be around second-hand cigarette smoke without fear of triggering my bowels to let go. That has changed, too, and even though I don't like the smell of tobacco since I quit smoking, my bowels do not react to it. It makes no difference whether I eat a soup and salad for a meal or a steak and bread; my bowels process the meals with regular, well-formed stools in about 24-hours.

My IBS is cured and no longer merely managed, yet I try to continue to maintain the healthy living habits I picked up along the way while trying to manage IBS. My long journey of enduring the symptoms and flare-ups, pain and embarrassment, and restricted lifestyle paid off big time because I kept trying new things to help my condition. I finally convinced myself that I could and would cure IBS, and I did it without the help of doctors and prescriptions. As far as I know, doctors don't think IBS can be cured, only managed even today in 2018. I have never bragged to any doctors that I cured my IBS because I did not want any negation of my accomplishment. I will always remember how the doctor I told about my IBS for the first time reacted with a sneer saying if I just quit smoking cigarettes and drinking coffee, it would go away. This was in the 1980s, but they still don't seem to know much about it today.

Finally

I waited years after the symptoms of IBS disappeared from my body before first writing this book because I wanted to make sure the cure was real. After seven years, I was certain enough to share my story and success with you. Now, as I write this update in 2018, I continue my free life without IBS and my bowels are even stronger and more reliable. I always wanted to share my journey with readers who are suffering with the disease like I did for thirty years. When I had IBS, symptoms would lessen and then get worse over and over again, and it was always there and appeared unexpectedly until my determination to cure myself paid off after I took matters into my own hands and found the two main things that made all the difference for me.

Even though doctors don't believe there is a cure and cannot really pinpoint a specific cause for the motility problems associated with IBS, you can try the things in this book, especially the final three: psyllium, probiotic dark chocolates, and L-glutamine along with a normal, healthy lifestyle (or any lifestyle you may lead, actually) to see if my cure works for you, too. I no longer need to take these things because I am confident IBS is gone and will never return. Feel free to let me know if these methods help you by contacting me through the publisher. The book seller will forward your email or letter to me. I would like to hear about your success and maybe share other success stories in future editions of this ebook.

I notice that there are many other books about IBS, and most are written by those researching the illness without really experiencing it. Many are filled with tedium that can distract you from finally curing yourself by exploring my successful two major methods or those you find on your own. I recommend that you avoid those researched books that repeat the same things about <u>managing</u> IBS. The only books on IBS worth reading are those written by sufferers who cured themselves or were cured somehow telling their own experiences firsthand. By all means, read those firsthand accounts by former sufferers for a cure for IBS to learn what might work for you. Don't merely manage the symptoms; cure the disease and be free from IBS. It is possible to cure IBS.

SUMMARY OF IMPORTANT POINTS

This list of important points and actions can help you to recall the actions I took to cure my IBS, which was almost entirely diarrhea/loose stools for decades.

- Begin with a diagnosis from a doctor to make sure you don't have a more serious problem in the digestive system. A stool sample should be given. However, you can always start with the two things that helped me first. If they don't help, definitely check to see if other medical issues exist.
- If the doctor says it is IBS, <u>delay</u> taking any normal medications they would prescribe to lessen symptoms. Taking them could make matters worse if you want to self-cure. However, do follow any dietary changes recommended if they help you manage symptoms until you cure the disease. Also, if an infection or parasite like bacteria/yeast/giardia/etc. is found in the stool sample, take the medications prescribed to kill the infection.
- Think back to when you began having symptoms of IBS to discover a root cause like drinking bad water in Mexico. If you can't make any connections to a causal event, that is okay.

- Take functional dark chocolates with probiotic bacteria daily for six months or less, as long as needed. It helped me the first week, so you may not need to take it too long. Take L-Glutamine as long as needed, too. I took it a few months, daily, then periodically.
- When symptoms of IBS go away, introduce trigger foods into your diet, like strong caffeinated coffee, spices, raw veggies, etc.
- Maintain healthy eating patterns like eating yogurt, veggies, fruit, whole grains, etc., since that is good for overall health. I eat all kinds of food without problems, including comfort foods and sweets without any problems. I try to keep a majority of my food as healthy as possible with veggies daily, but I also eat fast food, rich food, spicy food, meats, and somewhat unhealthy foods without any IBS symptoms.
- I no longer need functional chocolate or L-Glutamine since my bowels are strong, healthy, and without IBS symptoms of any sort, even when I drink strong coffee daily and eat sugary donuts occasionally.

Epilogue for 2018

A few years ago, I was in a casual conversation with a deli worker at a local supermarket buying some fried chicken. The middle-aged woman began telling me that she had IBS and the types of medications she was taking to manage symptoms so that she could work daily without problems. I thought about how odd it was to have this conversation while buying food she had prepared for the deli case because it was thoroughly unappetizing. Even though I wanted to let her know about my self-cure, it was too public a place for that, so I did not. I did not stop going to the deli after that, though, and I felt a little guilty not trying to help her. I realized that the personal journey of self-healing is one an individual takes on herself or himself. I'm sure there are other individualized ways to accomplish healing of this disease based on how it started. The important thing is to experiment to see what works for the individual before drowning in prescribed medications that only address symptoms. I like natural methods that restore my body to its normal functions in the gentlest way and not just manage symptoms of disease. We all want to live freely and happily without worry or embarrassment.

I have learned a great deal online from reading reviews and experiences of those who try different methods to help themselves, and I made it a point to try methods I felt might help to resolve a problem or help me to maintain health. Often, these things don't work or make any difference, but I tried them knowing that sometimes things do work or help my individual body, like L-Glutamine. I tried that only after reading a footnote in passing about how colon cancer patients use this to restore the bowel tissue damaged during treatment, etc. Follow your instincts with the positive mindset that you will cure yourself and the information and tools you need will come to you. Your own journey may differ from mine since the cause of your IBS might be different from mine. Good luck as you explore and experiment with the things you feel might help you cure IBS in addition to those two major things that made an almost immediate and permanent difference for me.

Contact me with questions and success stories, or write your own book about your own success story to help others. I would like to see all those researched books about <u>managing</u> IBS symptoms that exploit sufferers' desire for a normal life without the disease be replaced with true stories of healing like mine to help us cure this mysterious diagnosis doctors give us because IBS is a catch-all disease name for abnormal bowel motility issues like IBS that have no discoverable causes that doctors can pinpoint. It really is up to you to follow your instincts about research you read and as you try different remedies with a positive mindset that you will cure your ailment. Listen to your body like a detective.

www.ingramcontent.com/pod-product-compliance
Lightning Source LLC
Chambersburg PA
CBHW071201220526
45468CB00003B/1104